3-PORT VS 4-PORT LAPAROSCOPIC CHOLECYSTECTOMY

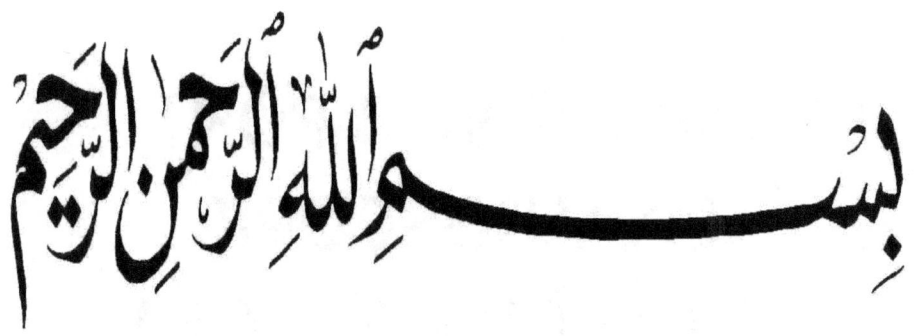

In the Name of Allah, the Most Gracious, the Most Merciful.

3-PORT VS 4-PORT LAPAROSCOPIC CHOLECYSTECTOMY

<u>CONTRIBUTIONS</u>

THE PROJECT WAS A SUCCESS BECAUSE OF THE DEDICATED
CONTRIBUTION AND HARD WORK OF THE FOLLOWING TEAM MEMBERS:

HAMZA ZAHIDULLAH MOHAMMAD ZAI
SYED SHAHMEER RAZA
NAMRA KHALIL
SHAYAN QADIR
SAAD AYUB KHAN

ACKNOWLEDGEMENTS

All the praises and thanks to Allah Almighty who enabled us to carry out this project without any complications and in time.

This project would not have been possible without the help and support of a number of people. It is our privilege to express our heartfelt gratitude to our Head of Department, Dr. Bushra Iftikhar for enabling us to avail this golden opportunity to prepare a project and help us gain an experience that will brighten up and open up ways for our future of research.

Special recognition must be accorded to our project supervisor Dr. Hamid Hussain for his valuable input, able guidance, encouragement, undying patience, whole hearted cooperation and constructive criticism throughout the duration of our project. Moreover, his methods of teaching the different rules and principles of research methodology, epidemiology, biostatistics and the techniques of using SPSS equipped us with the tools required to complete this project.

A special thanks to Dr. Rooh ul Muqeem who helped us understand with patience and dedication, the basics of laparoscopic cholecystectomy, including the procedure and how to go on about the project of such magnitude.

Last, but not the least, we are truly grateful for the help provided by the staff of the surgical wards of Khyber Teaching Hospital and Lady Reading Hospital. They helped us in every way possible in filling us in with the details of patients from whom the data was collected, without which this project would have been incomplete.

TABLE OF CONTENTS

ABSTRACT

BACKGROUND: With new advances in the field of surgery, there have been made many amendments in the methods of laparoscopic cholecystectomy. Since the advent of laparoscopic cholecystectomy, the four port technique has been a standard option for surgeons but for the past few years the role of the fourth trocar has been debated and three port techniques is sought to take its place.

OBJECTIVES: This study is an experimental prospective study which has been carried out to compare and contrast four port and three port techniques in terms of patient outcomes such as pain, nausea, satisfaction, hospital stay and complications rate.

METHODS: Data was collected from seventy seven patients who underwent laparoscopic cholecystectomy. Convenient sampling was used and sample was stratified into two age groups. Postoperative pain, nausea, analgesic requirements and the number of days of hospital stay was assessed amongst the patient using the visual analogue scale (VAS). Post-OP complications were also assessed.

RESULTS: "Young adults" (20-44 years) were 40 in number while 30 patients fell under the "Older adults" group (45 years and above). In "younger adults" the pain score was 4.29 (SD: $\pm$ 1.62) for three port and 5.78 (SD: $\pm$ 1.21) for four port, mean nausea score was less for four port i.e. 1.33 (SD: $\pm$ 2.17) than for three port 2.32

(SD: $\pm$ 2.24), Mean postoperative stay for four port 2.00 days (SD: $\pm$ 0 .71) was slightly more than three port 1.58 days (SD: $\pm$ 0.76).

In the older age groups the mean pain scores were : 3.33 (SD: $\pm$ 1.92) and 5.13 (SD: $\pm$ 1.46) for three and four port techniques respectively, mean nausea score amongst the old patients was not much different for three port and four port i.e. 1.40 (SD: $\pm$1.88) and 1.27 (SD: $\pm$2.09), patient satisfaction for three port 9.33 (SD: $\pm$ 0.97) was a little higher than four port 8.00 (SD: $\pm$ 1.22), mean postoperative stay for 3 port patients was 1.2 days (SD: $\pm$ 0.41) and for the 4 port patients was 1.8 days (SD: $\pm$ 0.56).

CONCLUSION: Three-port had a significantly better outcome than four-port technique in terms of post surgical pain, hospital stay and patient satisfaction. There was no significant difference in the complications rate and nausea.

PROJECT PROPOSAL

INTRODUCTION

Cholecystectomy is the surgical removal of the gallbladder for indications such as acute and chronic cholecystitis, biliary colic, cholelithiasis etc. The surgical techniques employed for the purpose are:

1) Open surgical intervention (an older and more invasive technique which exposes the patient to more risks as it involves a large incision) and

2) Laparoscopic cholecystectomy (in which a tiny camera is inserted and special surgical instruments are utilized to remove the gall bladder through small keyhole sized incisions), which is currently the most acceptable and widely used procedure.

Laparoscopic cholecystectomy (**Figure 2**) was first introduced by Philippe Mouret in France in 1987 and later established by Dubois and Perissat in 1990. Though, it has been subjected to several modifications over the years, laparoscopic

cholecystectomy is widely considered the gold standard in the surgical treatment of gallbladder disease.

Since the initial days, the standard laparoscopic cholecystectomy has employed four trocars (a trocar is a sharp edged medical instrument used to introduce into body cavities or blood vessels etc, endoscopes or instruments for such surgical procedures which require laparoscopic assistance)(**Figure 1**). The fourth (lateral) trocar is utilized to hold the fundus of the gallbladder in order to expose the Calot's triangle [5]. With newer refined techniques and better surgical skill and experience, it is now possible to carry out the procedure with a reduced number of ports and the fourth trocar may not be required.

Several studies have been carried out for the comparison of both, which conclude that the use of only three trocars is both feasible and safe [1] [2] [3] [9]. Though it may require a little more manipulation with instruments on the part of surgeon, the main advantages of the three port technique is the lesser degree of pain felt and analgesic dose required by the patient postoperatively [4] [6] [7] [8]. With just three port wounds, the patient recovers earlier and the postoperative hospital stay is reduced. Furthermore, the patient enjoys cosmetic benefit from the three-port technique [9].

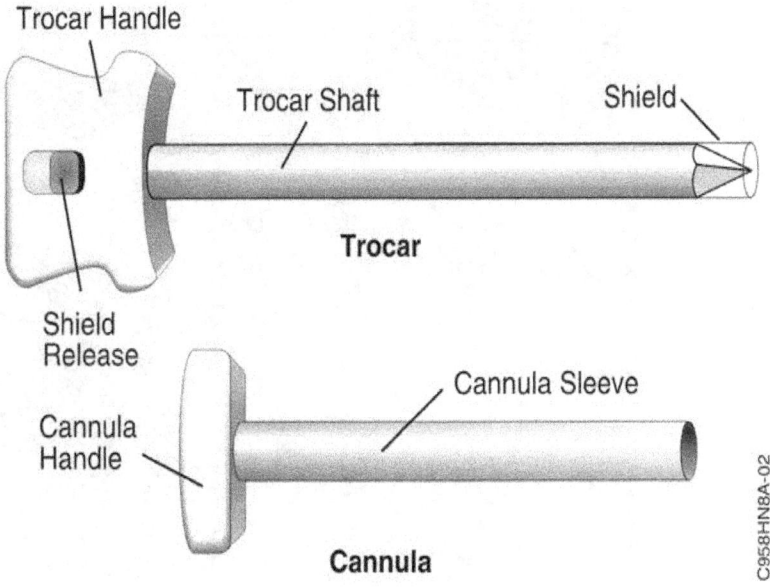

Fig. 1 Trocar

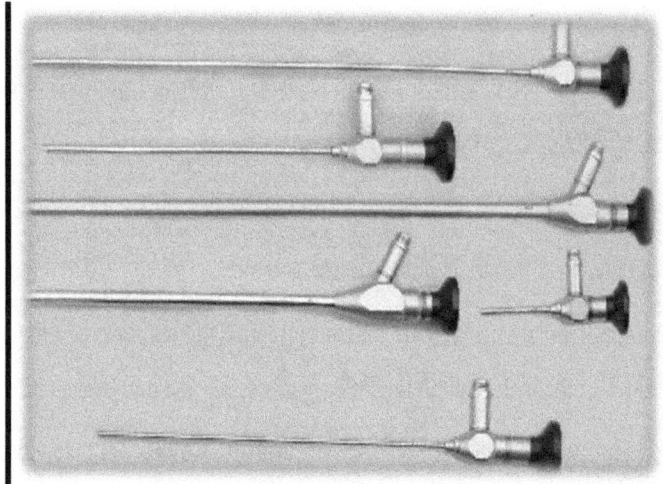

Fig. 2 Different sizes of Laparoscopes

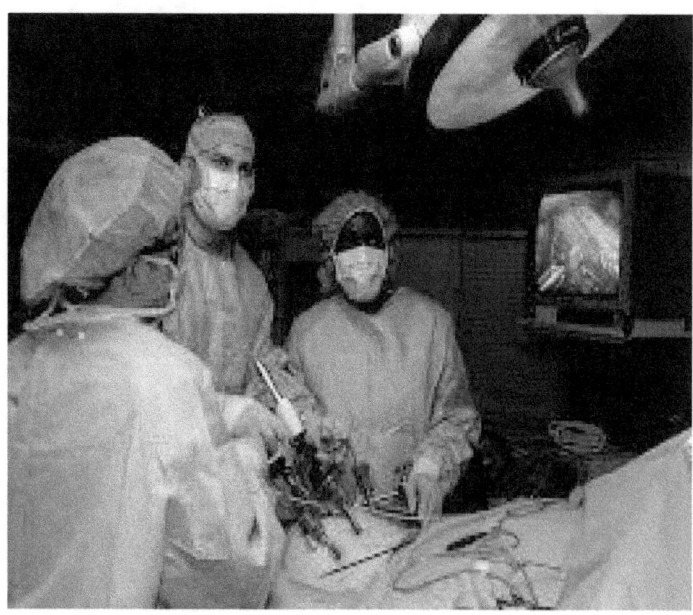

Fig. 3 Laparoscopic cholecystectomy in progress

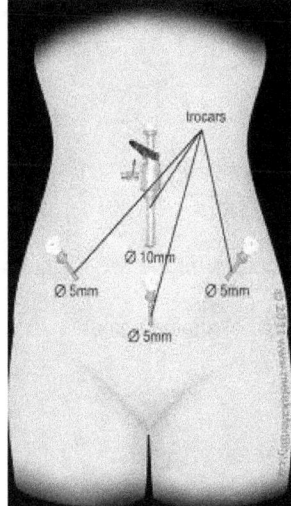

Fig. 4 Standard 4 port technique

RATIONALE FOR THE PROJECT

Even though many studies have been carried out, the benefits and harms of four

port and three port laparoscopic cholecystectomy in comparison to each other

are uncertain. That very question to determine which method is better in terms of

pain and nausea scores and giving overall better satisfaction to the patient is the

main drive behind our quest for undertaking this research in two tertiary care

hospitals Khyber Teaching Hospital and Lady Reading Hospital in Peshawar.

HYPOTHESIS

After reviewing past studies we are inclined to hypothesize that with less number of

incisions the patient outcomes may improve in terms of pain , nausea, satisfaction and hospital stay i.e. 3 port technique might prove better than the standard 4 port method.

OBJECTIVES

To assess the patient outcomes for the two methods in terms of:

1) Pain scores on VAS (Visual analog scale)

2) Nausea scores on VAS

3) Patient satisfaction score on VAS

4) Hospital stay in days/hours.

METHODOLOGY

- **Study Design**: Experimental Prospective study.
- **Sampling Technique**: Non-Randomized Convenient Sampling.

The patients were included in the study on the basis of availability, indifferent to the fact whether they underwent three or four port surgery. Due to this, randomization could not be carried out. However, the sample was divided into two strata based on the age of the patient. This helped to minimize the effect of confounding factor of age to affect the results of the study.

- **Sample size:** a total of 77 patients were recruited.

Out of this sample of 77, 7 patients were excluded from measuring outcomes in terms of pain, nausea, satisfaction and hospital stay. The reason for this was the conversion of these subjects from laparoscopic to open cholecystectomy.

- **Area of study:** Lady Reading Hospital, Peshawar (LRH) and Khyber Teaching Hospital, Peshawar (KTH)

- **Time of study:** Four months from March 2013 to June 2013

- **Target Population:** All patients indicated for laparoscopic cholecystectomy at KTH and LRH.

- **Consent:** All patients signed informed consent for the procedure and the follow-up study.

- **Stratification:** The first group included patients in the ages "18-44" while the second included patients in the ages "≥ 45".

- **Inclusion Criteria:** All male and female patients indicated for laparoscopic cholecystectomy at KTH and LRH.

- **Exclusion Criteria:** The exclusion criteria included patients who developed complications resulting in the procedure being turned into an open cholecystectomy.

- **Explanation of technique**

All procedures were carried out in accordance with the accepted protocols and by skillful specialist surgeons who were well experienced with both procedures. After routine preoperative work-up and administration of general anesthesia, the patients were subjected to their respective laparoscopic procedure. For the 4-port procedure, an 11-mm infraumbilical port, a 10-mm subxyphoid port and two 5-mm subcostal ports were used. In the 3-port laparoscopic cholecystectomy, an 11-mm infraumbilical port, a 10-mm subxyphoid port and a single 5-mm subcostal port was utilized. An operating telescope was inserted via the infraumbilical port. The gallbladder was retracted with long grasping forceps via the subcostal port and the cystic duct and artery were clipped. Dissection was carried out from the subxyphoid port and after changing the position of the operating telescope, the gallbladder was retrieved from the infraumbilical port. Wound dressings and surgical adhesive tape was applied to close the port site wounds and the post-surgical assessment carried out afterwards. The patients were put on postoperative antibiotics and given analgesics to control the pain.

- **Recording of Outcomes**

Our primary objectives were to determine the pain and nausea scores at 24 hours, postoperative stay in days and patient satisfaction at the time of discharge. The pain and nausea scores were evaluated using 10 cm visual analog scales given in **figure 5** (0 - none, 10 - extremely severe) by independent observers. The number of days in postoperative stay for each patient was noted and they were assessed for patient satisfaction at time of their discharge with VAS (0 - extremely dissatisfied, 10 - extremely satisfied). Secondary outcome measures to be noted were the need for use of surgical drains placed in the patients near the end of the procedure, and the complications rate for each procedure, both during surgery and postoperatively.

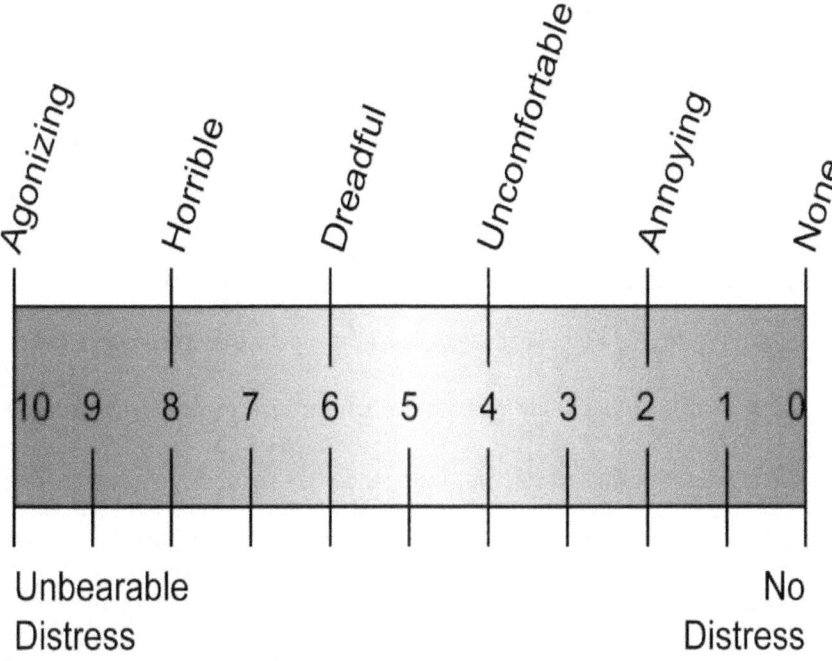

Fig. 5 Visual Analogue Scale (VAS)

- **Statistical Analysis**

The student T- test was used to evaluate the significance of each parameter. A p-value <0.05 was considered statistically significant. Statistical Package for Social Science (SPSS) Version 16 (Windows) was used for statistical analysis.

LITERATURE REVIEW

There were a limited number of studies that addressed this comparison. A study carried out in Nepal by Kumar et al helped us a lot in getting an overview of the topic in discussion [9]. In that study seventy five consecutive patients who underwent elective laparoscopic cholecystectomy were randomized to undergo either the 3-port or the 4-port technique. Four surgical tapes were applied to standard 4-port sites in both groups at the end of the operation. All dressings were kept intact until the first follow-up 1 week after surgery. Postoperative pain at the 4 sites was assessed on the first day after surgery by using a 10-cm un-scaled visual analog scale (VAS). Other outcome measures included analgesia requirements, length of the operation, postoperative stay, and patient satisfaction score on surgery and scars. Their results suggested that 3-port laparoscopic cholecystectomy resulted in less individual port-site pain and similar clinical outcomes with fewer surgical scars and without any increased risk of bile duct injury compared with 4-port laparoscopic cholecystectomy.

Another study was carried out by Trichak in Thailand in which 200 consecutive patients undergoing elective LC for gallstone disease were randomized to be treated via either the three- or four-port technique [1]. Their results were however a bit different in the way that they found no significant difference in other variables apart from the fact that 3 port patients consumed fewer amounts of analgesic injections (Nalbuphine). However they also concluded that three-port technique is as safe as the standard four-port one for LC. The main advantages of the three-port technique are that it causes less pain, is less expensive, and leaves fewer scars.

Other studies that that were reviewed did not compare the 3 and 4 port technique but they did however help us get a better understanding of the topic. They were:

1) Laparoscopic cholecystectomy: an original three-trocar technique [2]
Abstract:

At present, laparoscopic cholecystectomy is the treatment of choice for gallbladder stones. The operating technique reported by most authors includes the use of four trocars. We report a group of 710 consecutive patients treated by an original three-trocar technique. The use of the fourth trocar was necessary in only 55 cases (8%). However, among 56 cases of acute cholecystitis the use of the fourth trocar was necessary in 14 cases (25%) (*p-value* <0.01). Twenty-six laparoscopies were converted to open procedures (3.6%). Four common bile duct injuries were observed (0.5%): two of them among the 655 operations with three trocars (0.3%) and two after application of the fourth trocar at the beginning of the procedure because of dissection difficulties. Our results are similar to those using the "classic" four-trocar technique. Moreover, this technique is less expensive and allows one less scar.

2) **Pain after micro laparoscopic cholecystectomy** [3]

Abstract:

Background: Laparoscopic cholecystectomy (LC) is traditionally performed with two 10-mm and two 5-mm trocars. The effect of smaller port incisions on pain has not been established in controlled studies.

Methods: In a double-blind controlled study, patients were randomized to LC or cholecystectomy with three 2-mm trocars and one 10-mm trocar (micro-LC). All patients received a multimodal analgesic regimen, including incisional local anesthetics at the beginning of surgery, NSAID, and paracetamol. Pain was registered preoperatively, for the first 3 h postoperatively, and daily for the 1st week.

Results: The study was discontinued after inclusion of 26 patients because five of the 13 patients (38%) randomized to micro-LC were converted to LC. In the remaining 21 patients, overall pain and incisional pain intensity during the first 3 h postoperatively increased in the LC group (n= 13) compared with preoperative pain levels (p < 0.01), whereas pain did not increase in the micro-LC group (n= 8).

Conclusions: Micro-LC in combination with a prophylactic multimodal analgesic regimen reduced postoperative pain for the first 3 h postoperatively. However, the micro-LC led to an unacceptable rate of conversion to LC (38%). The micro-LC instruments therefore need further technical development before this surgical technique can be used on a routine basis for laparoscopic cholecystectomy.

3) **Mini-laparoscopic cholecystectomy vs. laparoscopic cholecystectomy** [4]

Abstract:

Background: We set out to assess the safety and efficacy of mini-laparoscopic cholecystectomy (MLC) in uncomplicated situations.

Methods: MLC was performed on 30 consecutive selected patients (<60 years old, ASA I-II, uncomplicated cholecystectomy) with one 12-mm and three 3-mm ports. The total operating time, conversion rate, degree of postoperative pain, duration of postoperative hospital stay, complications, and cosmetic results were all reviewed and compared with 30 cases of consecutive conventional laparoscopic cholecystectomy (LC).

Results: None of the patients in either group required conversion to open cholecystectomy. No complications were observed. The operating time and duration of hospital stay were similar in both groups. The level of postoperative pain was lower in the MLC group ($p < 0.001$). More patients in the MLC group expressed satisfaction with the cosmetic result ($p < 0.05$).

Conclusions: MLC was shown to be feasible in uncomplicated situations. Furthermore, it was associated with less pain and produced better cosmetic results than conventional LC. Randomized studies are still needed to confirm these findings.

4) The laparoscopic breakthrough in Europe [5]

Abstract: In the late 1980s, laparoscopy was essentially a gynecologist's tool. One of the French private surgeons, Phillipe Mouret of Lyon, shared his surgery practice with a gynecologist and thus had access to both laparoscopic equipment and to patients requiring laparoscopy. In March of 1987, Mouret carried out his first cholecystectomy by means of electronic laparoscopy. Although he never published anything about this experience, the news on his technique reached Francois Dubois of Paris. Although having no prior laparoscopic experience, Dubois acted immediately. He borrowed the instruments from gynecologists, performed his first animal experiments and, in April 1988, carried out the first laparoscopic cholecystectomy (LC) in Paris. Inspired by Dubois, Jacques Perissat of Bordeaux, introduced endoscopic cholecystectomy in his clinic and presented this technique at a SAGES meeting in Louisville in April 1989. Very soon, news of the French work in LC, soon, swept beyond the country's borders. Dubois and Perissat spoke enthusiastically about their work at the meetings and were largely responsible for establishing what is today called the French technique.

5) **Three-port micro laparoscopic cholecystectomy in 159 patients** [8]

Abstract

BACKGROUND:

Laparoscopic cholecystectomy has undergone many refinements including reductions in port size and number. This study attempts to determine whether further reduction in port size from that previously reported by us can reduce postoperative pain without compromising the efficacy of the surgery.

METHODS:

In this study, 159 patients underwent laparoscopic cholecystectomy with three ports: one 5-mm umbilical port, one 3-mm subxiphoid port, and one 3-mm port in the right subcostal position. Data were collected prospectively for each patient on the duration of analgesic use, quantity of analgesic tablets consumed, postoperative pain, most painful incision, and days of recovery required before return to activity and work. These measures were compared with those collected from a group of 100 patients who had undergone laparoscopic cholecystectomy with three 5-mm ports in a previous study.

RESULTS:

Patients in the current study group required analgesics for a longer duration (4 vs. 2.9 days; p = 0.001), used more analgesic tablets (10.7 vs. 8.1; p = 0.007), and reported greater postoperative discomfort (5 vs. 4.1; p = 0.016) as compared with all in the 5-mm port group. The 3-mm port group needed more days for recovery before leaving the house (2.9 vs. 2.7; p = 0.504), but they returned to work earlier (5.1 vs.

5.9; p = 0.065) than the group that had undergone cholecystectomy with three 5-mm ports, although there was not a significant difference between the groups. Operative time increased from 18.5 to 20.9 min (p = 0.054) in the group with two 3-mm ports. Five patients (3.1%) in the current group required enlargement of a port to complete the procedure, as compared with none in the comparison group. There was one complication (0.6%), as compared with two complications (2.0%) in the previous group.

CONCLUSIONS:

This study did not demonstrate a reduction in postoperative pain or a consistent improvement in recovery when the port size was reduced at the subcostal and subxiphoid positions. It did, however, show that ports could safely be reduced in size without a negative impact on the surgeon's ability to perform a cholecystectomy. Reducing port size can be a tool in the surgeon's armamentarium for use in the attempt to optimize cosmetic results.

ANALYSIS AND RESULTS

The total number of patients who underwent laparoscopic Cholecystectomy was 77 out of which 9 were males and 68 were females. 7 patients underwent conversion to open cholecystectomy and were excluded from the study. The mean age of the patients was 41.14 (SD $\pm$ 11.63) years. The patients who fell under the age group of young adults (20-44 years) were 40 out of which 31 underwent three port and 9 underwent four port techniques. On the other hand 30 patients fell under the Older age group (45 years and above) out of which 15 underwent three port and 15 underwent four port technique.

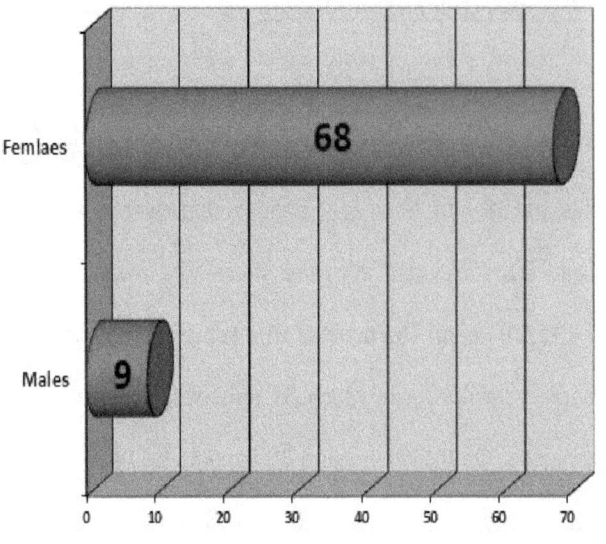

Gender Distribution

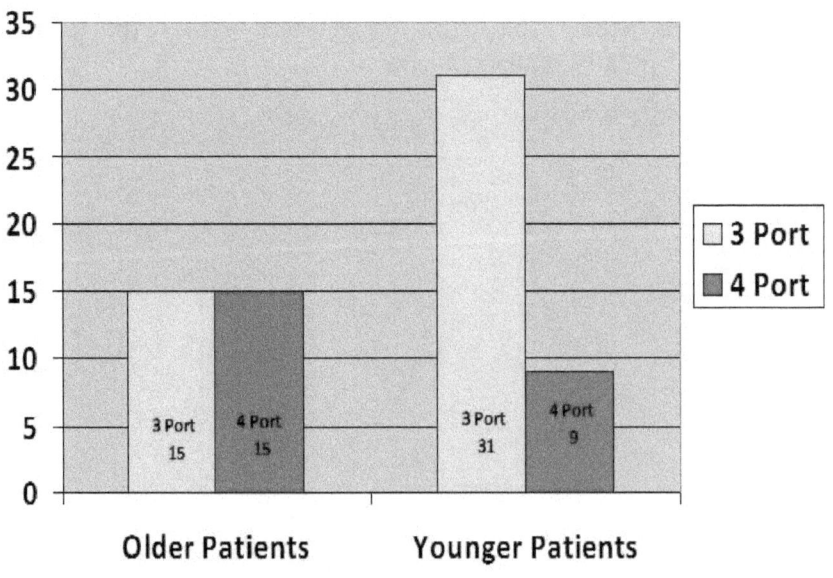

Older Patients   **Younger Patients**

Stratification of Sample

Younger Adults (18-44 years)

The mean pain score for three port technique was 4.29 (SD: $\pm$ 1.62) as compared to 5.78 (SD: $\pm$ 1.21) for four port. Mean nausea score among 3 port patients was 2.32 (SD: $\pm$ 2.24) while that of four port patients was 1.33 (SD: $\pm$ 2.17). Mean patients satisfaction scores at time of discharge was recorded as 9.04 (SD: $\pm$ 1.04) and 7.75 (SD: $\pm$ 1.38) for three port and four port patients respectively. Mean postoperative stay for the 3 port patients was 1.58 days (SD: $\pm$ 0.76) as opposed to that of 4 port patients that is 2.00 days (SD: $\pm$ 0.71).

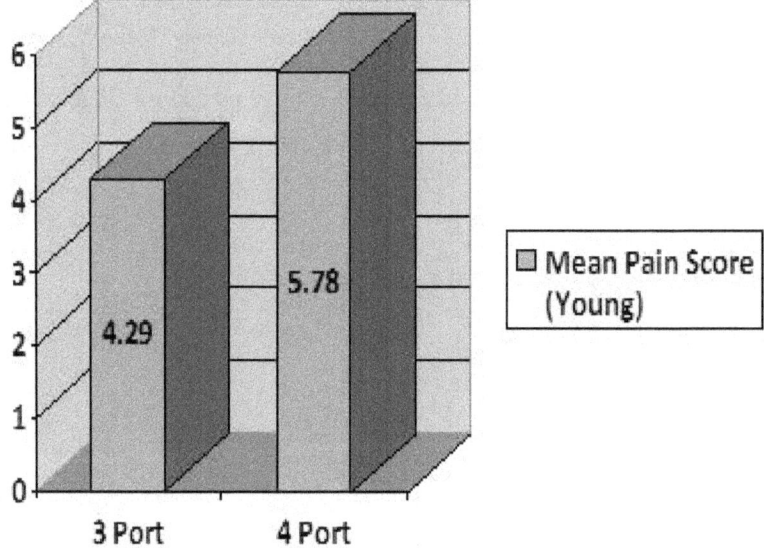

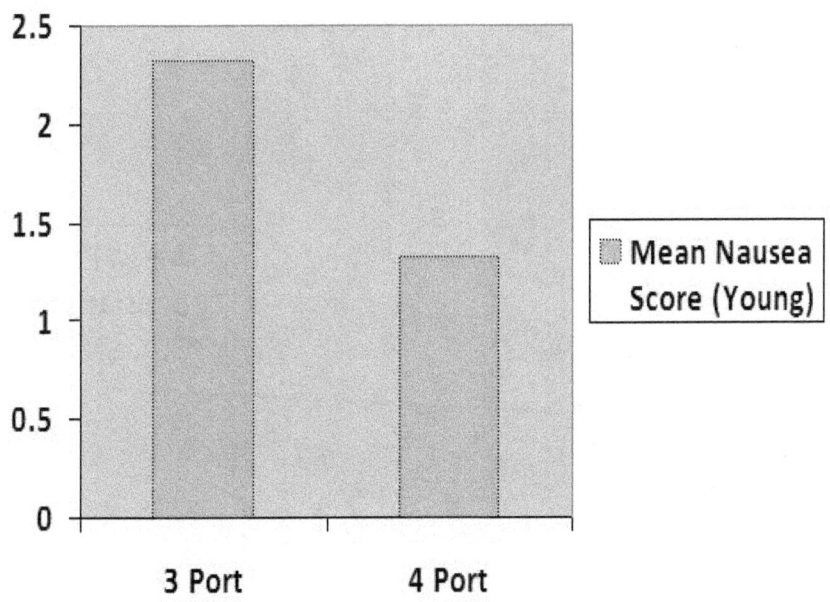

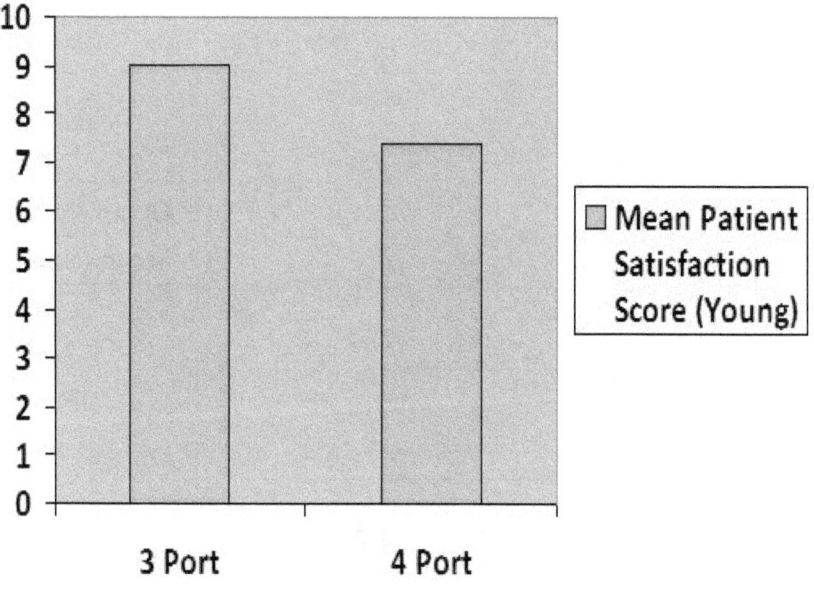

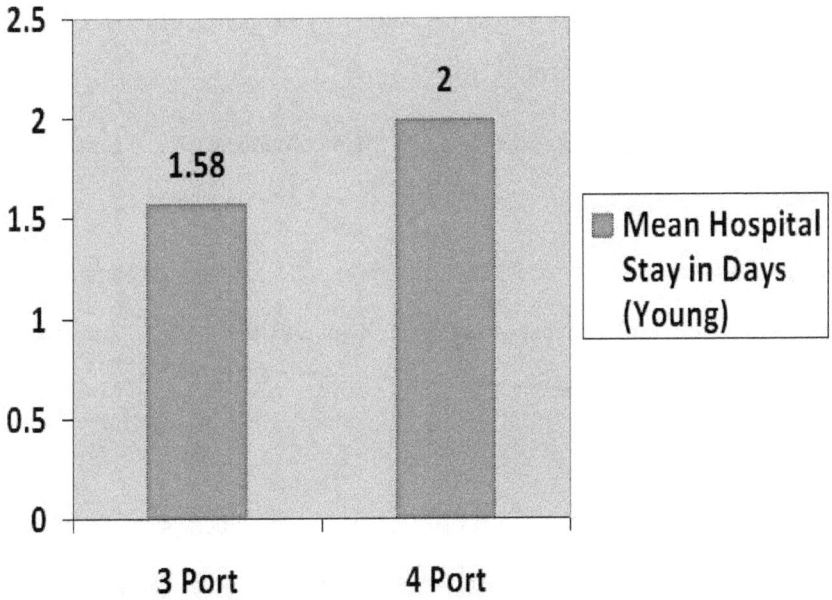

Older Adults (45 years and above)

The mean pain scores were: 3.33 (SD: ± 1.92) and 5.13 (SD: ± 1.46) for three and four port techniques respectively. Mean nausea score among 3 port patients was 1.4000 (SD: ± 1.88) while that of four port patients was 1.27 (SD: ± 2.09). Mean patient satisfaction scores at time of discharge for three port patients was 9.33 (SD: ± 0.97) and for four port 8.00 (SD: ± 1.2247). Mean postoperative stay for 3 port patients was 1.2 days (SD: ± 0.41) and for the 4 port patients was 1.8 days (SD: ± 0.56).

A significant correlation was established between the numbers of ports used and pain scores on VAS and patient satisfaction (p- Value < 0.05) in both the age groups.

Regarding the complications, 7 out of 77 patients (3 for 3-port, 4 for 4-port) of our inclusion sample had undergone conversion to open cholecystectomy; these were later excluded out before the statistical analysis of our results. Among the remaining 70 patients studied, three post surgical complications were reported for the 3-port procedure (one case each of port site bleeding, postoperative infection and gastrointestinal disturbance) and three complications reported for the 4-port procedure, i.e. two cases of port site bleeding and one of gastrointestinal disturbance.

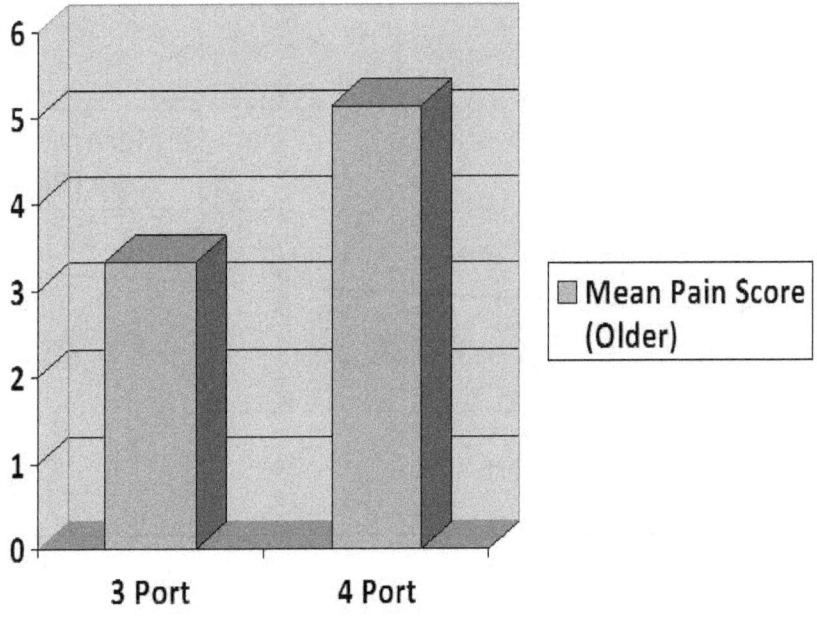

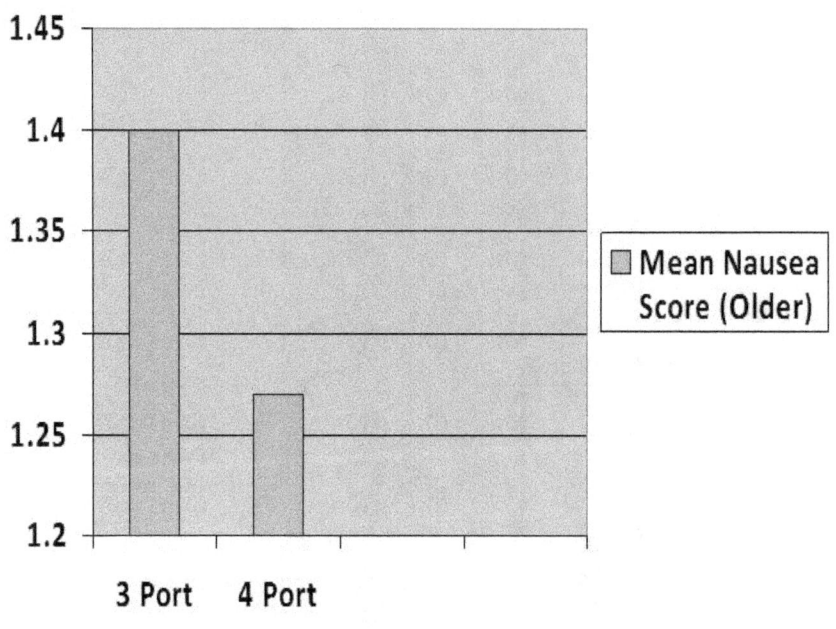

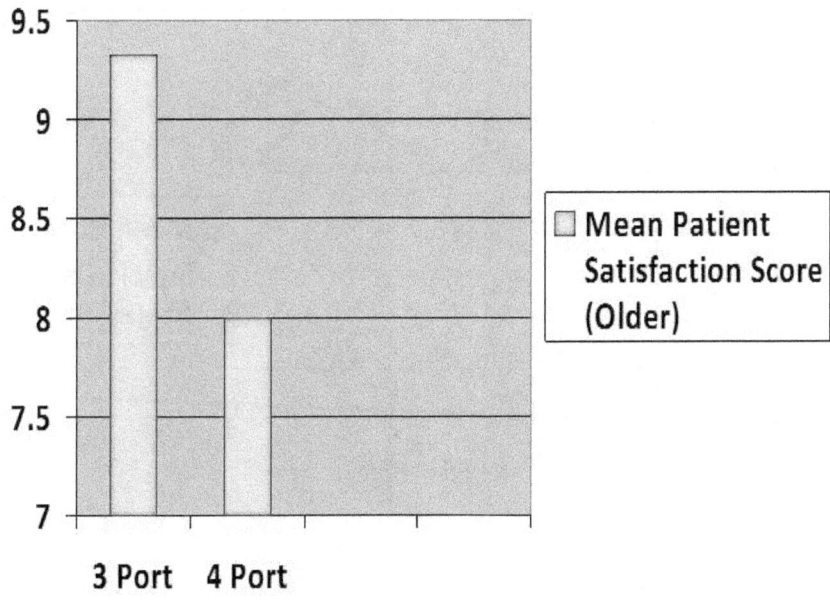

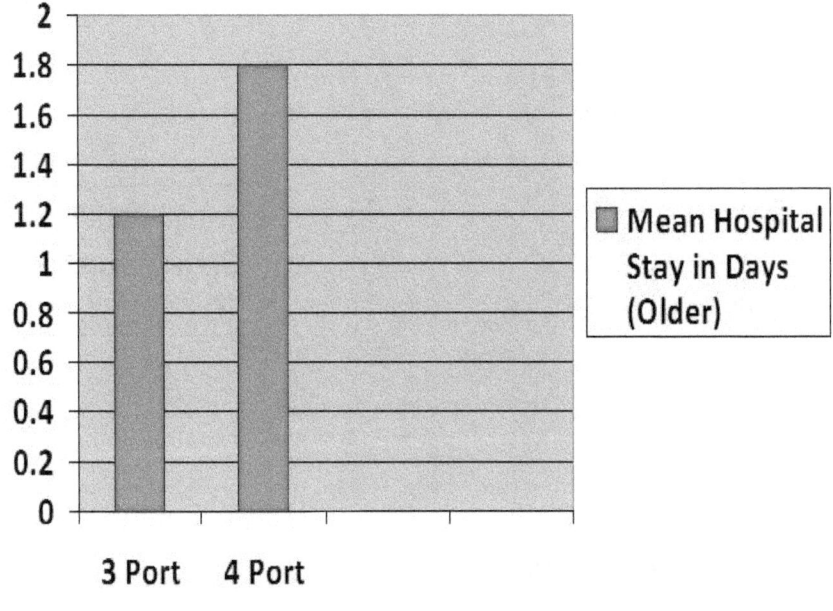

3 Port   4 Port

9%

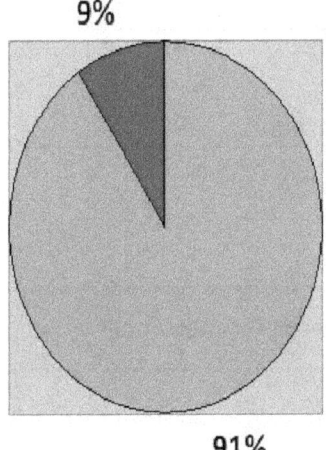

91%

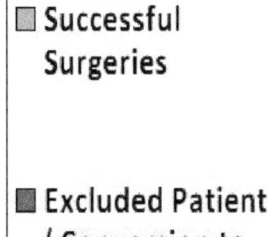

☐ Successful Surgeries

☐ Excluded Patients (Conversion to open cholecystectomy)

Procedure Used	Port Site Bleeding	Post-Surgical Infection	GIT Problems	Total
3 Port	1	1	1	3
4 Port	2	0	1	3

Comparison of Post-OP Complications

Results Summary for Younger Patients

	3 PORT	4 PORT	P-VALUE
Mean pain score on VAS	4.29 (SD ±1.62)	5.78 (SD ±1.21)	0.018
Mean nausea score on VAS	2.32 (SD ±2.24)	1.33 (SD ±2.17)	0.245
Mean patient Satisfaction score on VAS	9.04 (SD ±1.04)	7.75 (SD ±1.38)	0.009
Mean hospital Stay in days	1.58 (SD ±0.76)	2 (SD ±0.71)	0.000

Results Summary for Older Patients

	3 PORT	4 PORT	P-VALUE
Mean pain score on VAS	3.33 (SD ±1.92)	5.13 (SD ±1.46)	0.007
Mean nausea score on VAS	1.40 (SD ±1.88)	1.27 (SD ±2.09)	**0.856**
Mean patient Satisfaction score on VAS	9.33 (SD ±0.97)	8.00 (SD ±1.22)	0.004
Mean hospital Stay in days	1.2 (SD ±0.41)	1.8 (SD ±0.56)	0.000

DISCUSSION

The results of the study conducted were compiled and analyzed to determine the efficiency, safety and benefits of the two surgical techniques in terms of primary and secondary patient outcomes.

We found out that the 3-port laparoscopic cholecystectomy proved to be significantly better in terms of pain scores for both age groups. A mean pain score for the three port technique was 4.29 (SD: $\pm$ 1.62) for the younger patients and 3.33 (SD: $\pm$ 1.92) for the older patients whereas it was 5.78 (SD: $\pm$ 1.21) and 5.13 (SD: $\pm$ 1.46) for the younger and older 4-port patients respectively. A positive correlation was established between pain scores and the type of procedure in both age groups (p-value < 0.05). Two other studies carried out in Nepal and Ireland have also come up with the same association [9] [10]. Trichak, however, in his study carried out in Thailand concluded no such significant association.

Regarding nausea, the mean nausea score of 3 port patients was 2.32 (SD: $\pm$ 2.24) and 1.4000 (SD: $\pm$ 1.88) in young and elderly patients respectively. However, it was lesser in those patients who underwent 4 port surgery i.e. 1.33 (SD: $\pm$ 2.17) and 1.27 (SD: $\pm$ 2.09) in young and elderly patients respectively however this association was not statistically significant. Hence we can conclude that reducing the number of ports did not have any effect on the nausea felt by the patient. A significant correlation was also found out between nausea scores and pain scores on VAS in all patients of both groups (p- value < 0.05).

The hospital stay in days was also found to have a significant correlation (p-value < 0.05) with the procedure employed among both the age groups. We found that the mean postoperative stay among the younger adults for 3-port patients was 1.58 days (SD: ± 0.76) as opposed to that of 4-port patients that was 2.00 days (SD: ± .71). Among the older adults, mean postoperative stay for 3-port patients was 1.2 days (SD: ± 0.41) and for 4-port patients 1.8 days (SD: ± 0.56). Opting for the 3-port procedure proved to be more effective in terms of earlier discharge from the hospital and better recovery for the patient. Al-Azawi et al[10] also reports of a significance in the reduction of days of postoperative stay by opting for the 3-port procedure instead of the conventional 4-port one; mean postoperative stay, 3-port 2.8 days and 4-port 3.7 days, p-value = 0.005. Yet others, Trichak[1] and Chalkoo et al[11], maintain in their studies that both procedures yielded similar results and there was no significant association between the choice of the procedure and the postoperative hospital stay.

The satisfaction of the patients was also assessed in the study. It was observed that the mean patient satisfaction scores at the time of discharge for younger patients were recorded as 9.04 (S.D: ± 1.04) and 7.75 (S.D: ± 1.38) for three ports and four ports patients respectively. On the other hand, the scores observed for the older patients at the time of discharge were 9.33 (S.D: $\pm$ 0.97) and 8.00 (S.D: $\pm$ 1.22) for the three ports and four ports patients respectively. Moreover, comparing the patient satisfaction in terms of which hospital the procedure took place, the scores were 7.79 in Lady Reading Hospital (LRH) as compared to 9.26 in Khyber Teaching Hospital (KTH). The scores obtained from our study clearly suggests that the patient satisfaction was influenced by the number of ports involved in the procedure (p value= 0.05) Kumar et al[9] mentions in his study that the patient satisfaction for the 3 port (8.2 $\pm$ 1.7) and 4 port (7.8 $\pm$ 1.7) techniques are insignificant, (p-value= 0.24).

There were few post surgical complications during the stay after both the procedures. There were 3 patients who faced complications after the 3 port surgery i.e. one case each of bile leak, postoperative infection and gastrointestinal disturbance. Meanwhile, there was 1 case of gastrointestinal disturbance in the 4 port procedure.

CONCLUSION

Our study manifests clearly the benefits of three ports versus four port technique. Three port had a significantly better outcome than four port technique in terms of post surgical pain and patient satisfaction at time of discharge in both age strata.

Apart from that three port techniques seemed to improve, as compared to four ports, the mean number of days of hospital stay in both age groups. Three port technique however showed to have more postoperative complication rate than four ports but this did not reach any statistical significance.

RECOMMENDATIONS

Three port technique is as safe as the four port technique with less pain and hospital stay, more satisfaction and cosmetic advantages. We recommend surgeons to further pursue the safety and advantages of three port technique in their daily practice. We also urge the research opportunist surgeons and physicians to look more into the subject and document their findings as very few studies have been published relating this matter.

REFERENCES

1) Trichak S. Three-port vs. standard four-port laparoscopic cholecystectomy. Surg Endosc.2003; 17:1434–1436

2) Slim K, Pezet D, Stencl J Jr,Lechner C, Le Roux S, Lointier P. Laparoscopic cholecystectomy: an original three-trocar technique. World J Surg. 1995 May-Jun; 19(3):394-7

3) Bisgaard T, Klarskov B, Trap R, Kehlet H, Rosenberg J. Pain after micro laparoscopic cholecystectomy. A randomized double-blind controlled study. SurgEndosc. 2000 Apr; 14(4):340-4.

4) Sarli L, Costi R, Sansebastiano G: Mini-laparoscopic cholecystectomy vs laparoscopic cholecystectomy. SurgEndosc 2001, 15(6):614-8

5) Litynski G. Profiles in laparoscopy: Mouret, Dubois, and Perissat: the laparoscopic breakthrough in Europe (1987–1988). JSLS.1999; 3:163-167

6) Poon CM, Chan KW, Lee DW, et al. Two-port versus four-port laparoscopic cholecystectomy. SurgEndosc. 2003; 17 (10): 1624–1627.

7) Leggett PL, Bissell CD, Churchman-Winn R, Ahn C. Three-port micro laparoscopic cholecystectomy in 159 patients. SurgEndosc. 2001; 15 (3): 293–296.

8) Kumar M, Agrawal CS, Gupta RK. Three-port versus standard four-port laparoscopic cholecystectomy: a randomized controlled clinical trial in a community-based teaching hospital in eastern Nepal.JSLS. 2007 Jul-Sep; 11(3):358-62

9) Al-Azawi D, Houssein N, Rayis AB, McMahon D, Hehir DJ. Three-port versus four-port laparoscopic cholecystectomy in acute and chronic cholecystitis. BMC Surg. 2007 Jun 13; 7:8.

10) Indian J Surg. 2010 Oct; 72(5):373-6. doi: 10.1007/s12262-010-0154-9. Epub 2010 Nov 18. Is fourth port really required in laparoscopic cholecystectomy? Chalkoo M, Ahangar S, Durrani AM.

Fig. 1: http://www.fda.gov/ucm/groups/fdagov-public/documents/image/ucm197344.gif

Fig. 2: http://image.made-in-china.com/2f0j00sKhTHIUzVtbg/Laparoscope- Endoscope.jpg

Fig. 3: http://upload.wikimedia.org/wikipedia/commons/c/c3/Laparoscopic_stomach_surgery.jpg

Fig. 4: http://www.melakafertility.com/images/drawings/laparoscopy/lap-001.png

Fig. 5: http://cme.dannemiller.com/sections/professional/cme_article/images/EOP_pain-scale.jpg

APPENDIX

QUESTIONNAIRE

Patient Consent: *I agree to take part in the study that is designed with an aim to get a better understanding of the surgical techniques in use which will help to improve the health care standards of the society. I as a patient consent to the fact that the researchers can utilize my response in good faith to carry out their research*

_____*(Sign of patient)*_____

Date:

_____

Serial No.

_____

Name

_____

Age

_____

Sex

_____

Father's/Husband's Name

_____

Address

_____

Any past surgical history:

Yes___ No___

If yes, specify

_____

Any associated medical conditions (DM, HTN, IHD etc):

Yes___ No___

If yes, specify:

_____

Underlying pathology/Indication for surgery?

1. Acute cholecystitis

2. Chronic cholecystitis

3. Gallbladder stones

4. Asymptomatic patient with gallbladder stones at risk of complications.

5. Other

If other, Specify

_____

Surgical procedure: Laparoscopic

Cholecystectomy 4-ports___ 3-ports___

Complications during

surgery: Yes___ No___

If yes, specify_____

(Conversion to open surgery, bile duct injury, bile leak, bleeding)

Operation time in minutes

_____

Post-surgical pain assessment. (Score on VAS)

Score at 12 hours _____

Score at 24 hours _____

Post-surgical nausea (Score on VAS)

Score at 12 hours _____

Score at 24 hours _____

Analgesic requirement:

_____

Complications

Death of patient:

Yes___ No___

Post-surgical infection:

Yes___ No___

Post-surgical GIT problems:

Yes___ No___

Port site bleeding:

Yes___ No___

Post-operative stay (days)

_____

Patient Satisfaction at time of discharge

Score on VAS_____